Chronic Microvascular Ischemic Disease: Understanding the Condition and the Impact of Long COVID

Introduction:

Chronic Microvascular Ischemic Disease (CMVID) is a condition that affects the small blood vessels in the brain, leading to a range of neurological problems.

This disease primarily impacts older adults and is often associated with common vascular risk factors such as hypertension, diabetes, and high cholesterol.

The advent of the COVID-19 pandemic and the subsequent emergence of long COVID has added another layer of complexity to the understanding and management of CMVID.

This book delves into the origins, symptoms, diagnosis, and treatment of CMVID and explores how long COVID can exacerbate this already challenging condition.

Origins of Chronic Microvascular Ischemic Disease

CMVID is rooted in the concept of ischemia, which refers to a reduction in blood supply to tissues, causing a shortage of oxygen and nutrients needed for cellular metabolism.

In CMVID, this ischemia affects the brain's small blood vessels, also known as microvessels.

Over time, these vessels can become damaged due to various risk factors, leading to chronic ischemia and subsequent brain tissue damage.

<u>Key Risk Factors</u>

1. Hypertension:

 High blood pressure is one of the most significant risk factors for CMVID.

 Persistent hypertension can cause damage to the walls of small blood vessels, leading to narrowing or blockage.

 This restricts blood flow and results in ischemia.

2. Diabetes Mellitus:

 Diabetes can damage blood vessels through mechanisms such as inflammation, oxidative stress, and glycation of proteins.

 These changes make blood vessels more prone to narrowing and blockage, contributing to ischemia.

3. Hyperlipidemia:

 Elevated levels of cholesterol and other lipids in the blood can lead to atherosclerosis, a condition characterized by the buildup of plaques in the blood vessels.

 When this occurs in small brain vessels, it can significantly reduce blood flow.

4. Smoking:

 Smoking introduces various toxins into the body, which can damage blood vessels and promote inflammation and clot formation.

 This exacerbates the risk of ischemia in the brain's microvessels.

5. Age:

 As people age, their blood vessels naturally lose some of their elasticity and become more susceptible to damage.

 This age-related vascular decline can contribute to the development of CMVID.

<u>Symptoms of CMVID</u>

The symptoms of CMVID can vary widely depending on the extent and location of the brain tissue affected by ischemia.

Common symptoms include:

<u>Cognitive Impairments</u>

1. Memory Problems:

One of the earliest signs of CMVID is often difficulty with short-term memory.

Patients may struggle to recall recent events or conversations.

2. Executive Dysfunction:

 This includes challenges with planning, organizing, problem-solving, and multitasking.

 Individuals may find it hard to manage their daily tasks and responsibilities.

3. Reduced Mental Processing Speed:

 People with CMVID often experience slower thought processes, making it difficult to keep up with conversations or complete tasks quickly.

Motor Deficits

1. Gait Disturbances:

 CMVID can affect motor control, leading to unsteady walking, balance issues, and an increased risk of falls.

2. Fine Motor Skills:

 Tasks that require precise hand movements, such as writing or buttoning a shirt, can become challenging.

Emotional Changes

1. Depression:

 The impact of CMVID on the brain can lead to changes in mood, with depression being a common symptom.

2. Apathy:

 A lack of interest or motivation in activities that were previously enjoyed is another emotional symptom of CMVID.

Diagnosis of CMVID

Diagnosing CMVID typically involves a combination of clinical assessment and neuroimaging.

The goal is to identify the characteristic changes in the brain and correlate them with the patient's symptoms.

Clinical Assessment

A thorough clinical assessment involves evaluating the patient's medical history, risk factors, and presenting symptoms.

Cognitive tests may be administered to assess memory, executive function, and processing speed.

Motor assessments might include tests of balance and coordination.

Neuroimaging

Magnetic Resonance Imaging (MRI) is the primary tool used to diagnose CMVID.

MRI can reveal characteristic changes in the brain's white matter, often described as "white matter hyperintensities" or "leukoaraiosis."

These areas of increased signal intensity on T2-weighted images indicate regions of chronic ischemia and damage.

Treatment and Management of CMVID

There is no cure for CMVID, but managing the condition involves addressing the underlying risk factors and alleviating symptoms.

The approach is typically multifaceted, involving lifestyle changes, medications, and supportive therapies.

Lifestyle Modifications

1. Blood Pressure Control:

 Keeping blood pressure within a normal range is crucial.

 This can be achieved through a combination of medications, diet, and exercise.

2. Diabetes Management:

 Tight control of blood sugar levels helps prevent further vascular damage.

 This includes medications, dietary changes, and regular monitoring.

3. Cholesterol Management:

 Statins and other lipid-lowering medications can help reduce the risk of atherosclerosis and subsequent ischemia.

4. Smoking Cessation:

 Quitting smoking can significantly reduce the risk of further vascular damage and improve overall health.

5. Healthy Diet:

 A diet rich in fruits, vegetables, whole grains, and lean proteins, and low in saturated fats and sugars, supports vascular health.

6. Regular Exercise:

 Physical activity improves blood flow, reduces blood pressure, and supports overall cardiovascular health.

Medications

Medications may be prescribed to manage symptoms and address underlying risk factors.

These can include:

1. Antihypertensives:
 To control blood pressure.

2. Antidiabetic Medications:
 To manage blood sugar levels.

3. Statins:
 To lower cholesterol levels.

4. Antidepressants:
 To manage mood changes and
depression.

5. Cognitive Enhancers:
 To improve cognitive function
in some cases.

<u>Supportive Therapies</u>

1. Physical Therapy:
 Helps improve motor function and balance, reducing the risk of falls.

2. Cognitive Rehabilitation:
 Focuses on improving cognitive skills and compensating for deficits.

3. Occupational Therapy:
 Assists with daily living activities and adapting to physical limitations.

The Impact of Long COVID on CMVID

Long COVID, also known as post-acute sequelae of SARS-CoV-2 infection (PASC), refers to the persistence of symptoms long after the initial COVID-19 infection has resolved.

These symptoms can last for weeks, months, or even longer and can affect multiple organ systems, including the nervous system.

For individuals with CMVID, long COVID can pose additional challenges and exacerbate existing symptoms.

Cognitive Effects

Long COVID is associated with a range of cognitive impairments, often referred to as "brain fog."

This includes difficulties with memory, attention, and executive function.

For someone with CMVID, these cognitive challenges can be particularly debilitating.

The combined impact of CMVID and long COVID can lead to more pronounced memory problems, slower mental processing, and greater difficulties with planning and organizing.

Fatigue and Physical Health

Chronic fatigue is one of the most commonly reported symptoms of long COVID.

This persistent tiredness can significantly affect an individual's ability to carry out daily activities and participate in rehabilitation programs.

For patients with CMVID, who may already experience fatigue and decreased physical stamina, the added burden of long COVID-related fatigue can be overwhelming.

Motor Symptoms

 Long COVID can cause muscle weakness, joint pain, and other physical symptoms that exacerbate the motor deficits seen in CMVID.

 Gait disturbances and balance issues may become more severe, increasing the risk of falls and injuries.

Fine motor skills can also be further impaired, making everyday tasks even more challenging.

Emotional and Psychological Impact

 Both CMVID and long COVID can lead to emotional changes, including depression and anxiety.

 The psychological burden of dealing with two chronic conditions can be substantial.

Feelings of frustration, helplessness, and anxiety about the future are common.

Managing mental health becomes even more critical in this context.

Vascular Health and Inflammation

 COVID-19 is known to cause widespread inflammation and endothelial dysfunction, which can affect blood vessels throughout the body, including those in the brain.

 This inflammation can exacerbate the microvascular damage already present in CMVID, potentially accelerating the disease's progression.

The long-term effects of COVID-19 on vascular health are still being studied, but the potential for increased risk of ischemic events is a concern.

Managing CMVID in the Context of Long COVID

Managing CMVID in patients who also have long COVID requires a comprehensive and multidisciplinary approach.

It is essential to address both conditions simultaneously to improve the patient's overall quality of life.

Comprehensive Monitoring

Regular follow-ups with healthcare providers are crucial for monitoring the progression of both CMVID and long COVID.

This includes tracking cognitive and motor symptoms, as well as monitoring blood pressure, blood sugar levels, and cholesterol.

Adjustments to treatment plans should be made as needed to address new or worsening symptoms.

Symptom Management

1. Medications:

 Patients may require medications to manage cognitive symptoms, fatigue, and emotional health.

 Antidepressants and cognitive enhancers can be beneficial, as well as medications to manage physical symptoms such as pain and muscle weakness.

2. Physical Therapy:

 Ongoing physical therapy can help improve motor function, balance, and overall physical health.

 Tailoring the therapy to account for the additional fatigue and weakness associated with long COVID is important.

3. Cognitive Rehabilitation:

 Programs designed to improve cognitive function and compensate for deficits can help patients manage daily tasks more effectively.

4. Mental Health Support:

 Access to counseling and mental health services is essential for addressing the emotional and psychological impact of managing CMVID and long COVID.

 Support groups and therapy can provide valuable coping strategies.

Lifestyle Modifications

 Encouraging patients to adopt a heart-healthy diet, engage in regular physical activity, and maintain proper sleep hygiene is important for managing both CMVID and long COVID.

 Stress management techniques, such as mindfulness and relaxation exercises, can also be beneficial.

<u>Collaborative Care</u>

 A multidisciplinary team approach is often necessary to provide comprehensive care.

 This may include neurologists, cardiologists, physiotherapists, occupational therapists, and mental health professionals.

Coordination among these specialists ensures that all aspects of the patient's health are addressed.

<u>Conclusion</u>

Chronic Microvascular Ischemic Disease is a complex condition that affects the small blood vessels in the brain, leading to cognitive, motor, and emotional symptoms.

The emergence of long COVID has introduced additional challenges for individuals with CMVID, exacerbating symptoms and complicating management.

A comprehensive, multidisciplinary approach is essential for addressing the combined impact of these conditions.

Through regular monitoring, symptom management, lifestyle modifications, and collaborative care, patients with CMVID and long COVID can achieve better health outcomes and an improved quality of life.

Please use the next few pages
for your notes and debates.

www.ingramcontent.com/pod-product-compliance
Lightning Source LLC
Chambersburg PA
CBHW050828250726
48653CB00006B/2495